Contents

Introduction to
Kinesiology Taping
What is Kinesio?

By Amira Abdallah

Kinesio tapes, developed by the Korean Medical Association for Balancing Taping and produced in South Korea since 1997 Korean tapes are the best tapes on the world market, as judged by specialists and experts in the field of medicine and rehabilitation.

Uses of Kinesiology Taping

Tape Taping lends support and stability to muscles and joints. It optimizes pain relief care and Remodeling care without ever restricting normal body movement.   It is safe for all ages and skin types.

Not only does .....it offer the needed support for atheletes normal daily activities, but it also eliminates pain and tension associated with muscle and joint injuries or postural disorders. Because of the way it is crafted, the adhesive tape facilitates blood and lymphatic flow in the skin, which in turn contributes in reducing inflammation and again become a special new tool for medics in losing local fats and enhansing metabolism, so it helps fasting the rate of weight loss and encouraging our clients to fullfil his job

Main Uses

Injuries and their treatment

Providing assistance to vulnerable areas

Muscle re-education

Increasing performance

Scar Management

How it works

Creates space in joints

May change signals on pain pathways

May improve circulation of blood and fluids

How to apply

As a rule, lymph(perforated) tapes are glued without tension, with the exception of some cases.

After gluing, it is necessary to carefully smooth the tapes with the palm of your hand to activate the adhesive layer and more tightly to the skin. The application should not hinder movement; it can be left on the skin for 3-5 days. **Read the** complete

list of **BB LYMPH TAPE ™ Kinesiology Tape Guidelines** before performing drain **taping** .

General Rules of applying Kinesio tapes

How to Put Kinesiology Tape on

To apply the tape, remember these steps:

- Clean and dry the area first. Lotions and oils can prevent the tape from sticking.

- Trim excess hair. Fine hair shouldn't be a problem, but dense hair could keep the tape from getting a good grip on your skin.

- For most treatments, you'll start by tearing the backing paper in the center.

- Cut rounded corners at the ends of each strip if they don't already have them. The rounded corners are less likely to get snagged against clothing; and helps to keep the tape on longer.

-When you apply the first tab to anchor the strip, let the end recoil slightly after you take off the backing paper. You don't want any stretch in the last two inches at either end, because those tabs are just to hold the tape in place. If you stretch the ends, the tape will pull your skin, which could cause irritation or make the tape detach sooner.

- Keep your fingers on the packing paper to hold the tape. Touching the adhesive part will make it less sticky.

- Your therapist can let you know how much stretch to use in the treatment area. To get a 75 percent stretch, extend the tape as far as it will go and then release it about a quarter of its length.

-When you stretch the tape, use the whole length of your thumb across the tape to get an even stretch.

- After you apply the tape, rub the strip vigorously for several seconds. Heat activates the glue. Full adhesion usually takes around 20 minutes.

How to safely remove kinesio tape

If you use the tape for more than a few days, it may begin to loosen on its own. Here are

some *hints for removing the tape without damaging your skin.*

- To loosen the strip, use some oil (such as baby oil or olive oil) or lotion on top of it. - Take it out carefully.

- Don't pull. Don't try to pull up.

- Press pressure on your skin after pushing up one end of the strip to separate it from the tape.

- Instead of pulling the tape straight up away from you, pull it back against itself. Gently compress your skin while pushing the tape back toward the end tab.

- As you go, run your fingertips along your skin.   If your skin is irritated or damaged,... don't reapply tape.

- Consider talking...... talk to your physical therapist or doctor.

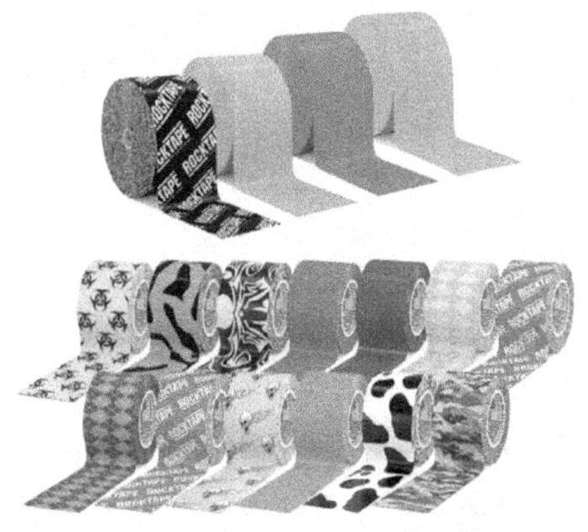

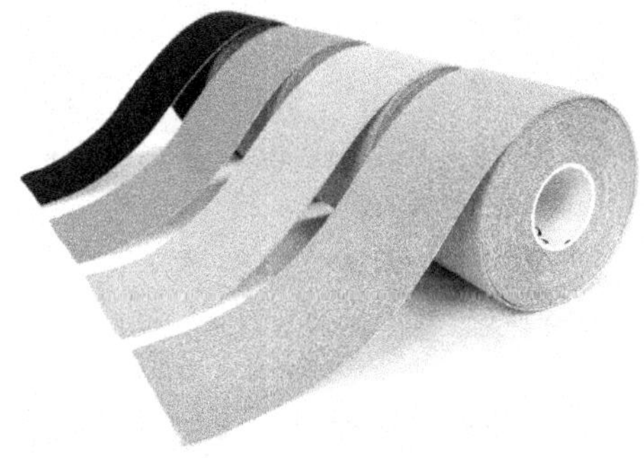

Never use Kinesiology in these situstions

- Wounds that have not healed. Putting tape over a wound might cause infection or skin damage.

- Deep vein thrombosis is a kind of thrombosis that occurs in the veins Increasing fluid flow might dislodge a blood clot, which could be deadly.

- Cancer is active. Increasing the blood supply to a malignant tumor may be hazardous.

- Lymph node removal is a surgical procedure that involves the removal of lymph nodes. Swelling may result from an increase in fluid where a node is absent.

- Diabetes. You may not detect a reaction to the tape if you have diminished feeling in some locations.

- Allergy. If your skin is sensitive to adhesives, you may get a severe response.

Skin that is easily broken. If your skin is prone to ripping, avoid using tape on it.

Size

There is a wide variety of kinesio tapes , differing in size colors materials

It should be noted that, depending on the characteristics, this or that type of kinesiotape has its own characteristics and scope. Therefore, in this book we will tell you in details about each type of tapes and types of injuries in which they are used.

The main characteristics that you should pay attention to when choosing tapes include:

·Kinesio tape in a roll of 5 cm * 5 m (roll width 5 cm, roll length 5 m) is the most common (standard) size of kinesio tape used by both athletes and traumatologists in the treatment of patients with injuries of the musculoskeletal system. The main types of pathologies in which such a tape is applied include: pain in the neck and shoulder girdle, back and lower back pain, sprains of the lower

extremities, "tennis elbow" and many others. By choosing a standard roll of kinesio tape, you can cut the strip to the length you need, depending on the area on which the applique will be glued. Usually one standard roll of 5 m length is enough for many applications. Also in our online store you can purchase an original face tape from South

KoreaBB FACE TAPE ™ **5 cm wide . This width is suitable** for most face and neck applications.

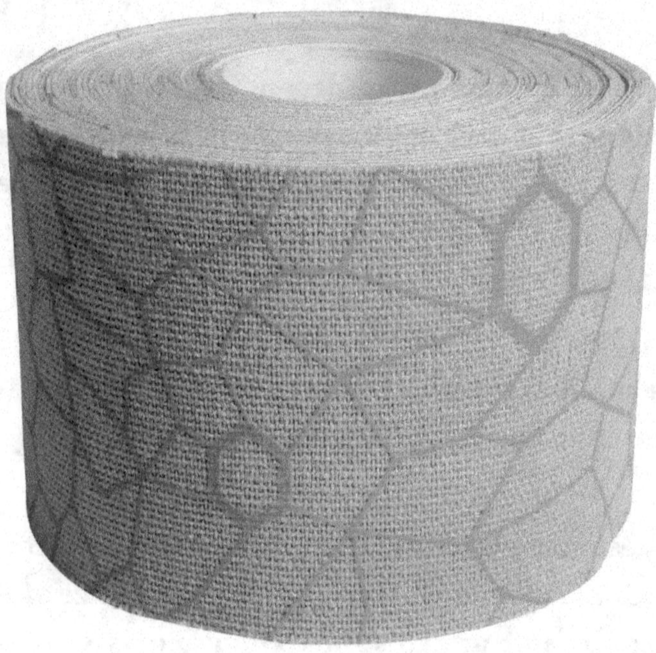

- **Roll 2.5 cm * 5 m** - the narrowest in the range of cotton kinesio tapes. They will be the best option when used on narrow parts of the body (for example, the phalanges of the fingers), when kinesio taping children and applying applications to the face and neck. For face taping, **BB FACE TAPE ™ 2.5 cm wide kinesiotape sets** , designed specifically for aesthetic taping,are best suitedwith detailed instructions for use inside each package.

- **Roll 3.75 cm * 5 m** - an ideal choice for applying on small-sized parts of the body, as well as in the face, neck area in cosmetology and during aesthetic taping procedures. Made of eco-friendly cotton with hypo-allergenic glue. The roll length (5 m) is enough for a sufficient number of applications.

- **Roll 7.5 cm * 5 m** - this width of the tape (7.5 cm) is ideal for applying on large injured areas of the body, as well as for taping with

- lymphedema and swelling of the knee joint. In addition, a tape of this size is widely used in plastic surgery to eliminate puffiness after surgery.

- **Roll 10 cm * 5 m** - like the previous type, tapes of this size are mainly used for application to wide areas of the body or for lymphatic drainage.

- **Rolls 17 m and 32 m long** - these tapes are a kind of standard tapes with the only difference that their length is longer. As a rule, such economical rolls (each of which is enough for more than 60 and 120 applications, respectively) are purchased by professional athletes or doctors who regularly use taping, as well as those who use tapes at home for a course of procedures. In addition, by purchasing rolls of 17 meters and 32 meters,

- you save and get several meters of tape for free!

- **Precut kinesiology tapes** - the area of application of such tapes is the same as that of standard kinesiology tapes. However, it is more convenient to use them, since each roll consists of twenty pre-cut strips with a length of 25 centimeters and different widths (5 cm, 7.5 cm or 10 cm). When taping, you do not need scissors, which is the main advantage of this type of tape. The disadvantages of this type include the fact that depending on the problem area on which the applique is applied, the tapes may not be enough, and you still have to cut the necessary applique from standard rolls.

Unfortunately, not all of types in the market are of high quality and meet the necessary requirements for elasticity and extensibility.

Most of the brands claiming origin from Germany, the Netherlands, the United States are actually manufactured in China, which is reflected in the quality of the cotton and the glue base. Due to the insufficient quality of the glue, *Chinese tapes adhere much worse to the skin*, fall off faster and can cause allergic reactions. Therefore, when buying, it is very important to clarify the country of origin of the tape and carefully read the production address indicated on the packaging, so as not to purchase low-quality products and not be disappointed in the effectiveness of the kinesio taping technique.

Kinesio tapes BBTape (Bio Balance Taping) are manufactured in <u>South Korea to the highest quality</u> standards

The assortment of the BBTape brand is currently the widest in the world and includes kinesio tapes in twelve different colors, as well as a collection with designer and children's colors. Let's put it bluntly that the color of the tape does not in any way affect its healing properties, but it has a certain physiological effect on the patient:

- brown - refers to neutral colors;
- blue - has a calming effect on the patient;
- pink - evokes positive emotions;

- yellow - promotes mental balance and harmony;
- Orange with Left - has a stimulating effect;
- black is the color of individuality;
- green - neutral, non-irritating look;
- red - stimulates the patient's desire for a speedy recovery.

Also, besides the usual colors, other tapes which are distinguished by modern prints, are great for

taping children and will undoubtedly attract the attention of others.

For taping in pediatrics, speech therapy, pediatric traumatology and rehabilitation .

Despite the skepticism of most people towards the color therapy method, doctors are still inclined to believe that the color of the tape plays an important role in the patient's recovery and helps to improve his emotional background.

Madicare®

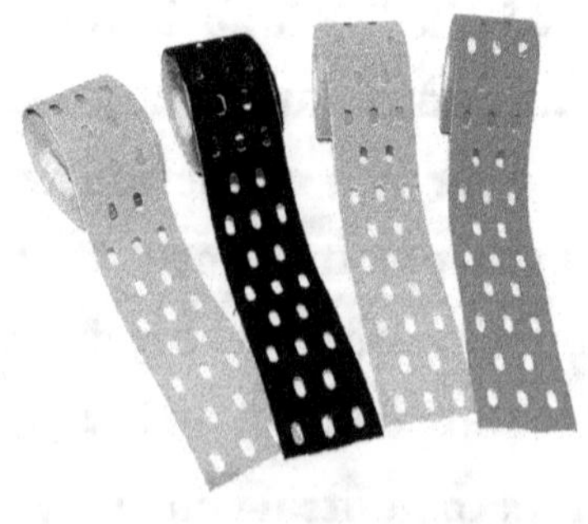

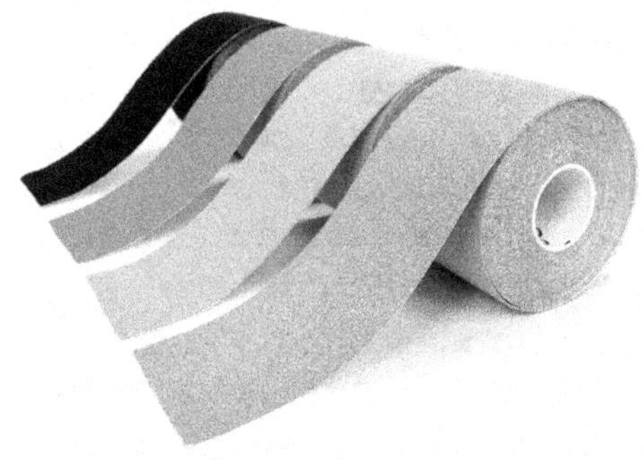

- **Cotton kinesio tapes** are the basic type, the characteristics of which are close to the properties and elasticity of human skin, and do not cause irritation. Such tapes consist of cotton covered with a special hypoallergenic acrylic glue, the properties of which are largely activated when the body temperature rises (for example, when rubbing the tape with your hand after applying an applique or during the training process). Ideal for face taping.

- **Nylon kinesiotapes** are distinguished by an increased level of elasticity compared to standard tapes, which makes them indispensable during an especially intense (with the use of heavy loads) training process. The peculiarity of such kinesiotapes is that when stretched, they store energy and release (direct) it in the relaxation phase - this contributes to a better flow of oxygen and nutrients to muscle tissues.

-

- **Nylon kinesio tapes**, unlike cotton ones, are capable of stretching not only in length, but also in width, which makes them indispensable for many clinical diseases and in hospital treatment.

- **Synthetic kinesio tapes (made of rayon) are distinguished by a thinner and more durable material, which ensures a snug fit of the tape to the skin and increases the wearing period. Fully breathable, moisture resistant and has a silky, tactile surface with a slight gloss. They have proven themselves in cosmetology, because ideal for sensitive areas (face, neck, chest) and in pediatrics when taping children.**
- **Kinesio tapes with reinforced glue - have good water resistance, which is why they are popular among athletes involved in water sports, as well as when taping areas of the body with increased sweating.**
- **Kinesio tapes with soft glue are ideal for taping**
- **people with particularly sensitive skin prone to**
- **allergic reactions, children, the elderly,**
- **as well as for use in neurology and pediatrics.**
-
-
- **Fluorescent kinesiotapes are cotton kinesiotapes with safe fluorescent paint applied to the surface of the tape. They are used mainly by athletes and amateurs when playing sports in the dark - for example, running in open areas, skiing, cycling, etc.**

Cross Tape (cross tapes)

Are small patches made of polyester, fastened together according to the lattice principle. The use of cross-tapes helps to improve the mobility of injured joints and tissues, as well as to significantly reduce pain. In addition, such a grid patch is successfully used to combat diseases of various internal organs, and its use in most cases is combined with standard taping. However, when applying cross tapes, it is necessary to know the main acupuncture and trigger points on the human body in order to achieve maximum effect.

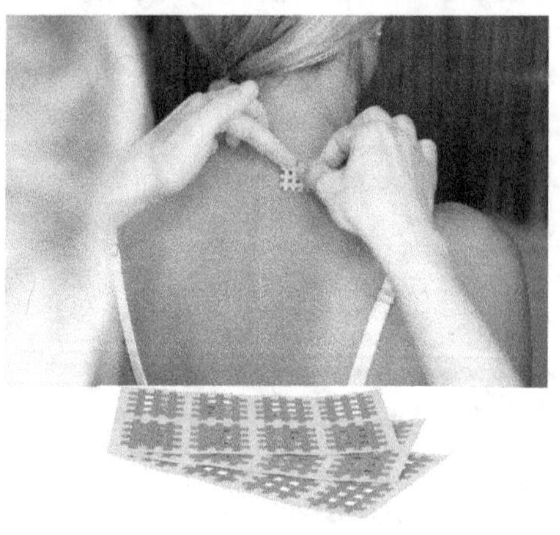

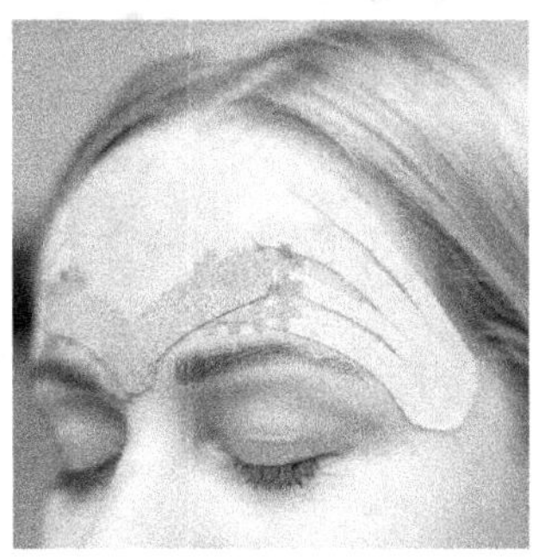

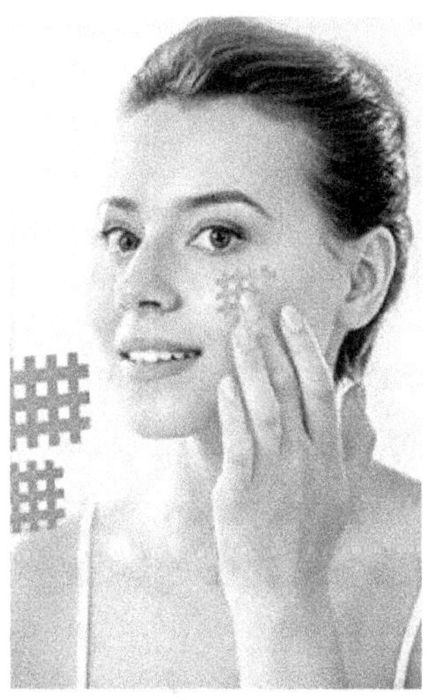

- the presence of a hypoallergenic adhesive composition;
- ease of use;
- compact size;
-
-
- good resistance to moisture, which is especially important

for water sports.

There are three sizes of cross tapes - 2.1 * 2.7 cm (size A); 2.8 * 3.6cm (size B); 4.9 * 5.2cm (size C). You can use any size depending on the area that the patch will be applied to. Alternatively, use the smallest cross tapes (A) for more precise blending. If you are in doubt about the choice of size or want to compare the effect of each one, you can immediately purchase a set of cross tapes , including all 3 values - A, B, C   for more tangible results.

In addition to cross tapes in the form of lattices, also there are a variety of them - aku tapes are polyester patches, but in a cruciform shape.

They are distinguished by their small size - 1 cm x 1 cm, due to which they are able to exert a point (acupuncture) effect in hard-to-reach areas of the face and body (corners of the eyes and lips, para-nasal sinuses, parotid region, neck, fingers, etc.).

The cross-taping technique is used for the following types of pathologies:

- painful sensations in various parts of the body (including headaches, menstrual pains, joint and muscle pains) and internal organs (cough, asthma, gastro-intestinal disorders);
- pain and disorders associated with an imbalance of joints, muscles and nerves;
- tension in muscle tissue;
- painful sensations in the joints after

undergoing surgery or excessive stress;

- circulatory disorders;
- various diseases of the musculoskeletal system;
- With swelling of the limbs or certain areas of the body.
- To support and increase the endurance of muscles

and joints, prevent new injuries.

Cross-taping is successfully combined with kinesiotaping, which results in faster and

<u>The advantages of BBTape cross tapes in comparison with kinesio and other types of tapes include:</u>

- effectively cope with pain in muscle and joint injuries and help restore the balance of the whole body;
- help to quickly remove traces of edema, bruises and bruises;
- effective for allergies and asthma, as well as for diseases of internal organs;
- Suitable for people with sensitive skin and for application to particularly sensitive areas such as face, neck, décolleté, etc.
- Due to its small size and lattice shape, the cross-tapes are comfortable to use, because almost not felt on the skin and do not attract the attention of others;
- cross-tapes can be worn on the skin for several days, however, due to the fact that cross-taping has an effect on the entire body, it is
-
- recommended to remove the applications if you feel dizzy or unwell;
- Cross tapes are completely breathable, which allows the skin to breathe, they are easy to stick on and feature high quality hypoallergenic glue.
- They are not afraid of moisture: in them you can calmly take a shower and do water sports.

Thus, cross-taping (cross-taping) is a very effective and universal taping technique based on the knowledge of oriental medicine, and is actively used by specialists around the world.

In accordance with Chinese medical doctrine, the healing effect of cross-taping is achieved due to the effect of the patch on the so-called meridians located under our skin and responsible for the circulation of energy in the human body.

So, in the event of any pathology, the energy flow is blocked and cross-tapes help restore its normal movement.

This is achieved due to the fact that when this special patch is applied, the skin is slightly lifted and the energy can flow unhindered in its usual way, which leads to the removal of pain and the restoration of the balance of the whole body.

At the same time, it is very important that only an experienced specialist who is familiar with acupuncture and who knows the location of myofascial trigger points on the human body can stick the cross-tapes. Also, before applying the cross-tapes, it is very important to conduct contact tests to accurately assess the initial state of the patient and determine the direction of the cross-

tape tapes. Otherwise, the desired result from the use of cross tapes may not be achieved.

In most cases, BB Cross Tape is applied to:

- pain points;
- trigger zones or points, which are areas of muscle that can cause pain in other parts of the body;
- acupuncture points, the impact on which normalizes the work of certain systems of the human body.

Thanks to the application of the cross tape to the above points, the circulation of blood circulation is normalized, as a result of which the desired effect is a

Unlike standard kinesio tapes , which are cotton or synthetic tape of various widths,

cross tapes are made of PVC (polyvinyl chloride) and have a fine-fiber structure. Usually cross tapes are available in three sizes (A, B, C) and are selected depending on the area to be applied. Cross tapes are not elastic and it is recommended to wear them no more than one day, unlike kinesio tapes. This is due to the fact that when applied correctly, cross-tapes can have a very powerful effect on the human body, changing thermoregulation and restoring the overall balance of the body.

The use of cross tapes is possible both as a separate type of treatment, including in cases where kinesio taping has shown low efficiency, and in addition to the kinesio taping technique or other methods to enhance the therapeutic effect. In some cases, cross-taping is used instead of kinesio-taping due to the more gentle effect on the skin (in

infants, people with sensitive skin, with a tendency to allergies, etc.).

Thanks to the application of the cross tape to the above points, the circulation of blood circulation is normalized, as a result of which the desired effect is achieved. Cross-taping affects the entire human body, not just the place where

pain is present or there is a disturbance caused by an imbalance of muscles / joints / nerves, and relieves pain, helping to restore the balance of muscles, joints and nerves.

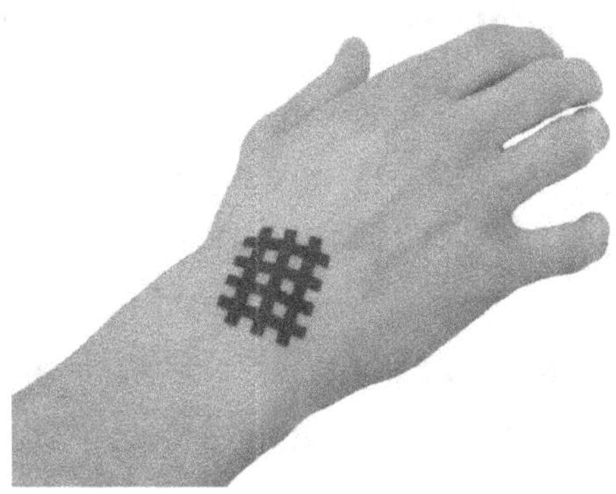

Perforated tapes

Are specially designed for *lymphatic drainage taping of the face and body.* Numerous studies carried out in South Korea have shown that the special perforated structure of the kinesio tapes promotes better stimulation of lymph flow and blood flow, so excess fluid and other metabolic products are more intensively removed from the tissues.

Lymph tapes for Face not only show better results in comparison with conventional tapes for lymphatic correction and elimination of edema, but also have a number of advantages. Perforation reduces the area of the adhesive coating,so these tapes can be used in sensitive areas of the face, neck and chest.

At the same time, they do not require preliminary cutting before carrying out lymphatic drainage, taping and better adhere to the skin.

Perforated Body Tapes have proven to be particularly effective against cellulite and subcutaneous fat. Thanks to the slotted structure, they provide maximum stimulation of the skin receptors, and allow you to achieve a high-quality lymphatic drainage effect, in the shortest possible time. Also, perforated tapes can be used on sensitive areas, of the body such as chest, abdomen and neck

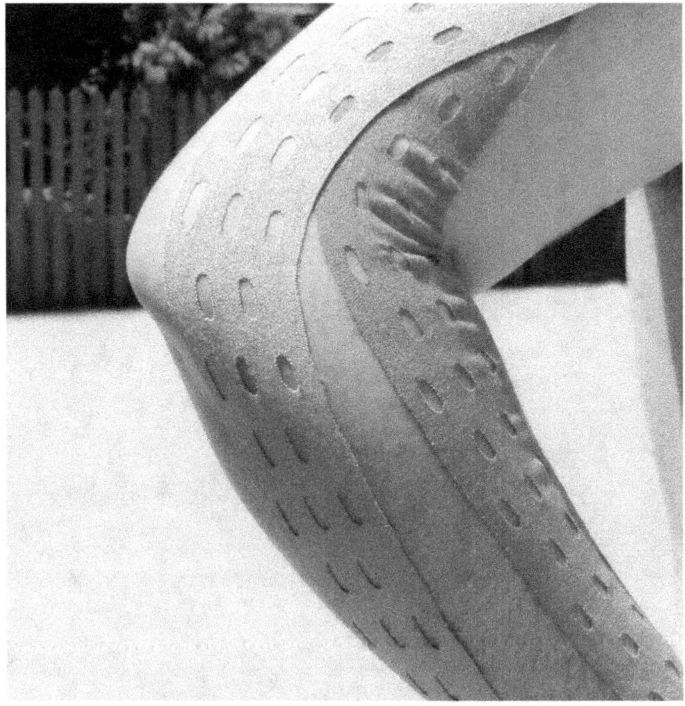

- **Losing weight,**
- **Sculpturing your body**
- **Treating ugly cellulite**
- **Boosting metabolism**

Flat Belly

Kinesiology Tapes may not be a quick way to lose weight, but it is the only way to target local areas, such as belly fats. It works by enhancing the lymphatic system and opening its pathways to flush the fats away. The second reason to get rid of fats (via Kinesiology Tapes) is by working on specific meridia to enhance metabolism.

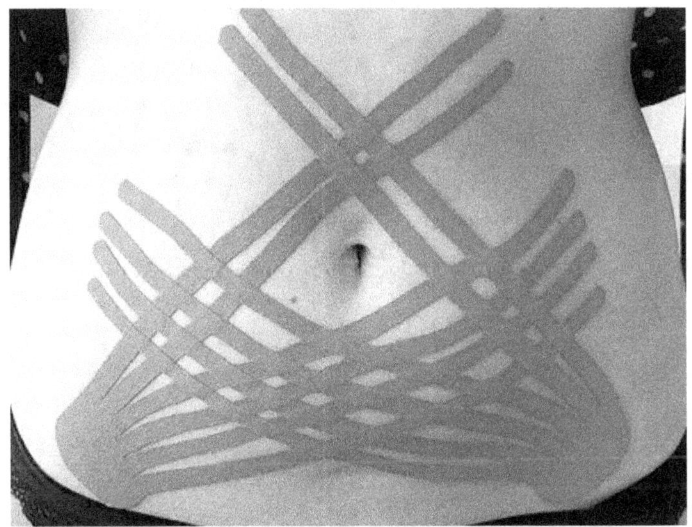

These two application patterns are aiming to lose weight from the belly and of course, cellulite will decrease too and the area below the belly button 5cm is the best place to boost metabolism for all the body and ease fats lipolysis.

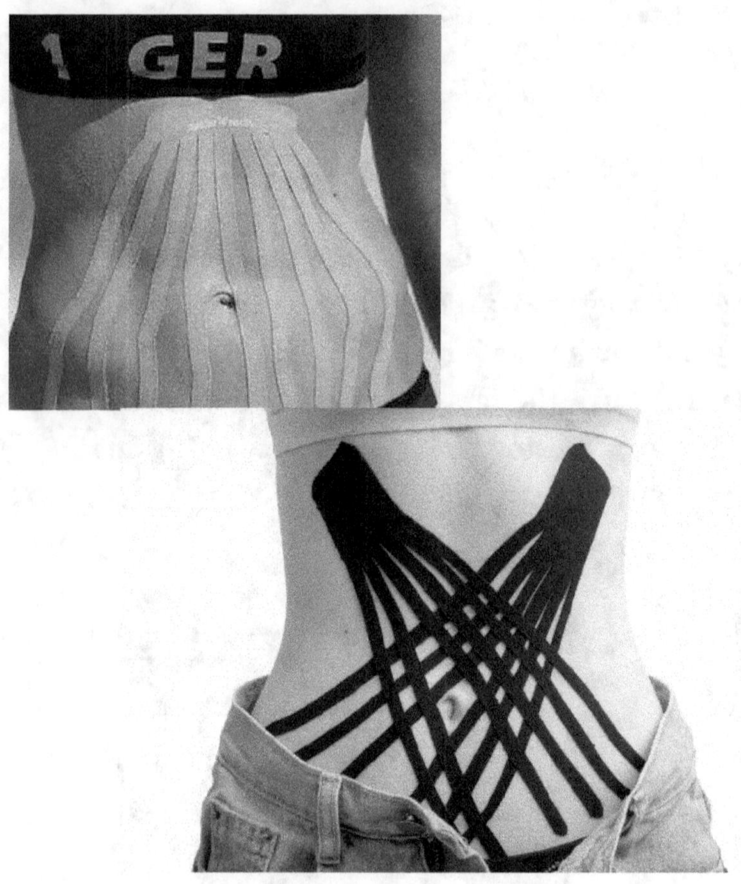

is aiming the lateral areas of the abdomen sides (love handles) and reducing the subcutaneous fat in this area by accelerating lymphatic drainage and removing excess fluid.

For this application, use **LITE Kinesio Tape for Sensitive Skin or standard Cotton Kinesio Tape 5 cm wide.**

Cut the kinesio tape 5 cm wide and 50-70 cm long into four pieces as a lymph tape, leaving 4-5 cm uncut at the base. For each side of the abdomen, you will need two appliqués cut in the same way.

The anchors (bases) of the tapes should be glued without tension to the area under the breast towards the lower part of the sternum.

Direct the ends of the first application of the tape along the front surface of the abdomen towards the thighs, as shown in photo the pink tapes. Stick the second application

of the kinesio tape on the problem areas on the sides, leading the tape towards the buttocks, as shown in photo the turquoise tapes.

Repeat the two applications on the other side in the same way.

Applications for lymphatic drainage are glued without tension. You can wear kinesio tapes for up to three to four days. Maximum efficiency is achieved with daily application changes.

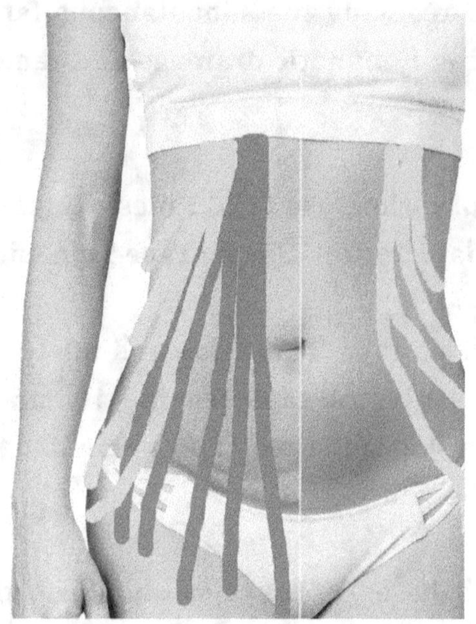

https://www.youtube.com/watch?v=CKlf_xVgW7s

Cellulite

is the dimpled-looking skin that commonly occurs in the thigh region. It forms when fatty tissue deep in the skin pushes up against connective tissue. It's estimated that more than 85 percent of all women 21 years and older have cellulite, so its merely a combination of random colonized fibrous tissue clogged with a lot of subcutaneous fats

In order to eliminate them both you should boost and un-clog your LYMPHATIC S and let it do the hole job, The perforated tapes works very well to open and boost your lymphatic system, just put it in the right way and position

For the abdominal area apply it like the photo on the left with 25% stretching, let it for 5 days and 2 days off for 3 months.....only you should drink lot of water(14 glasses/ day) with a low fat diet,

If you don't have perforated tapes do as the application on the photo on the right, 5 days and 2 off for 3 months

Madicare®

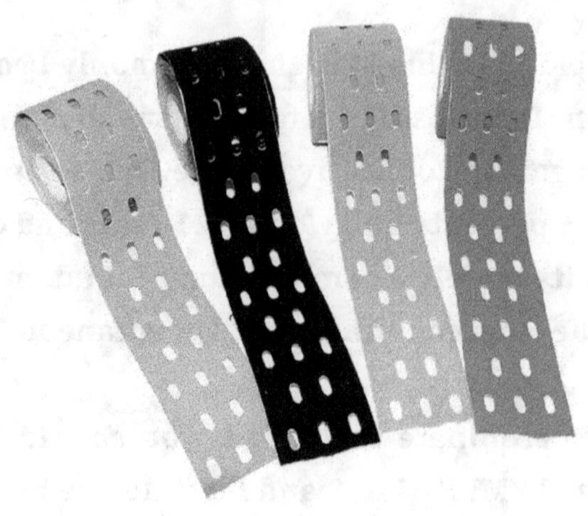

Cellulite is the dimpled-looking skin that commonly occurs in the thigh region. It forms when fatty tissue deep in the skin pushes up against connective tissue. It's estimated that more than 85 percent of all women 21 years and older have cellulite, so its merely a combination of random colonized fibrous tissue clogged with a lot of subcutaneous fats

In order to eliminate them both you should boost and un-clog your LYMPHATIC S and let it do the hole job, The perforated tapes works very well to open and boost your lymphatic system, just put it in the right way and position

For the abdominal area apply it like the photo on the left with 25% stretching, let it for 5 days and 2 days off for 3 months.....only you should drink lot of water(14 glasses/ day) with a low fat diet, If you don't have perforated tapes do as the application on the photo on the right, 5 days and 2 off for 3 months

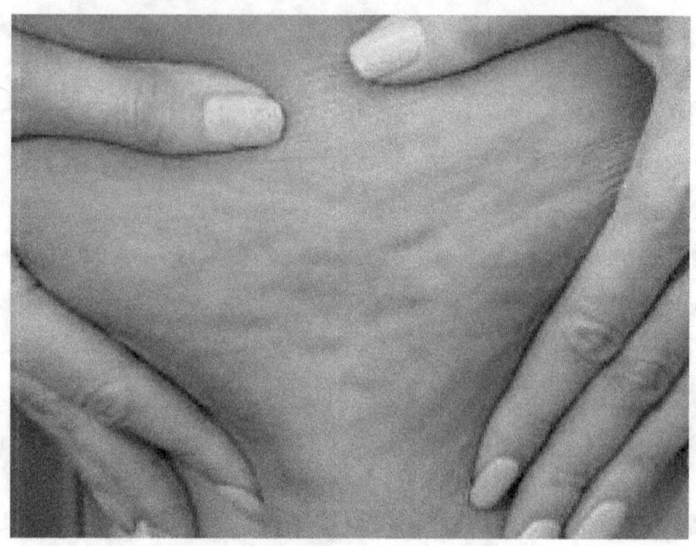

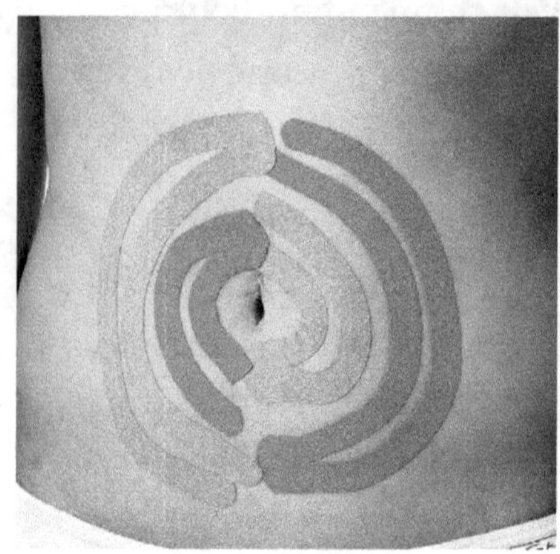

the Rectus Abdominus muscles

are largely affected

After pregnancy and having a baby

those kinesio applications are giving good results in treating rectus Diasthesis, we do th pattern for 5days and 2days off for at least 2months and then we try to strengthen the abdominus recti muscles with the

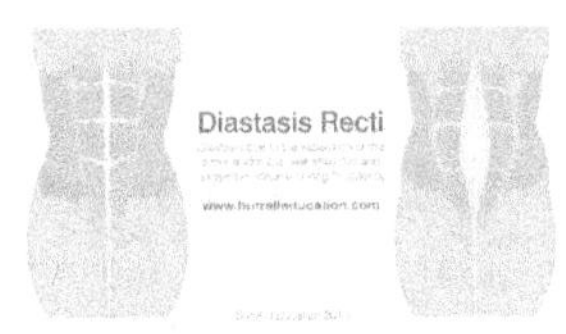

four patterns also with regular exercise

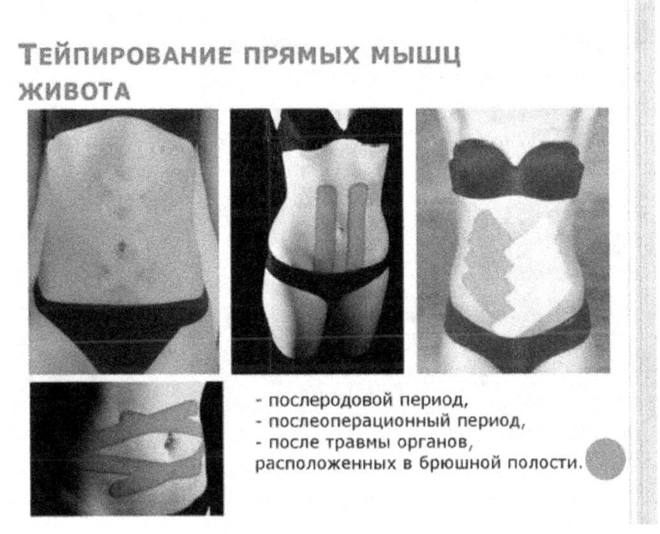

Boosting Metabolism

We use Kinesio to stimulate or awake certain points on our skin according to the Chinese old medicine, In traditional Chinese medicine, each acupressure point on the body exists on an energy pathway called a "meridian." These meridians are named according to the various organs in the body.

Each acupressure point along a meridian is named using the letters corresponding to that meridian, followed by the location of the point on the pathway. These acupressure points also have corresponding traditional names.

In the upper picture an example of tapinging to stimulate some abdominal points

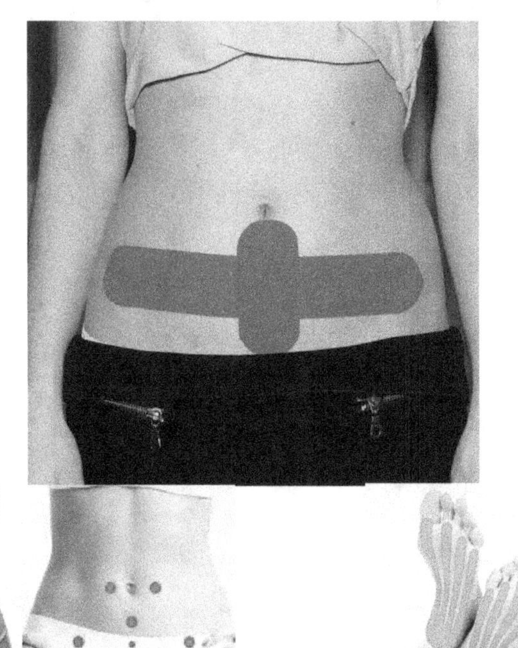